Digest This Now!

Liz Cruz, M.D.

Best Selling Author of "Answering the Call" &
Tina Nunziato, Certified Holistic Nutrition Consultant

Digest This Now! by Liz Cruz, M.D. & Tina Nunziato, C.H.N.C

Published by www.drlizcruz.com
9515 W. Camelback Road, Ste. 102
Phoenix, AZ 85037

Cover design by Natalie Goebig.

This book is not intended to provide medical advice or to take the place of medical advice and treatment from your personal physician. Readers are advised to consult their own doctors or other qualified health professionals regarding the treatment of their medical problems.

Neither the publisher nor the authors take any responsibility for any possible consequences from any treatment, action or application of medicine, supplement, or preparation to any person reading or following the information in this book. If readers are taking prescription medications, they should consult with their physicians and not take themselves off of medicines to start supplementation without the proper supervision of a physician.

International Standard Book Number:
978-0-9916138-0-9 (paperback)

Contents

This book is dedicated to you – because without you, there would be no reason for it!

We are so excited to finally deliver this amazing information into your hands.

There were so many times Tina and I wanted to bury this information and move on but you: our patients, clients, friends and family kept encouraging us to push on.

Thank you!

Acknowledgements

We'd like to thank our Mothers Elizabeth Cruz, Sr. and Karen Nunziato who repeatedly took care of our children while we wrote this book.

We'd also like to thank all of our friends and associates who helped us edit this book – especially Phil Tompkins, our personal-development guru, for spending so much time getting into the nitty-gritty with us.

A special shout out to our girl Natalie Goebig for helping us design an amazing cover for the book in addition to designing the new look for DrLizCruz.com and the DNA for Digestive Health – you are an amazing graphic designer and friend.

Finally, we would like to thank God for continuing to guide us and remind us how important it is to rely on Him for everything.

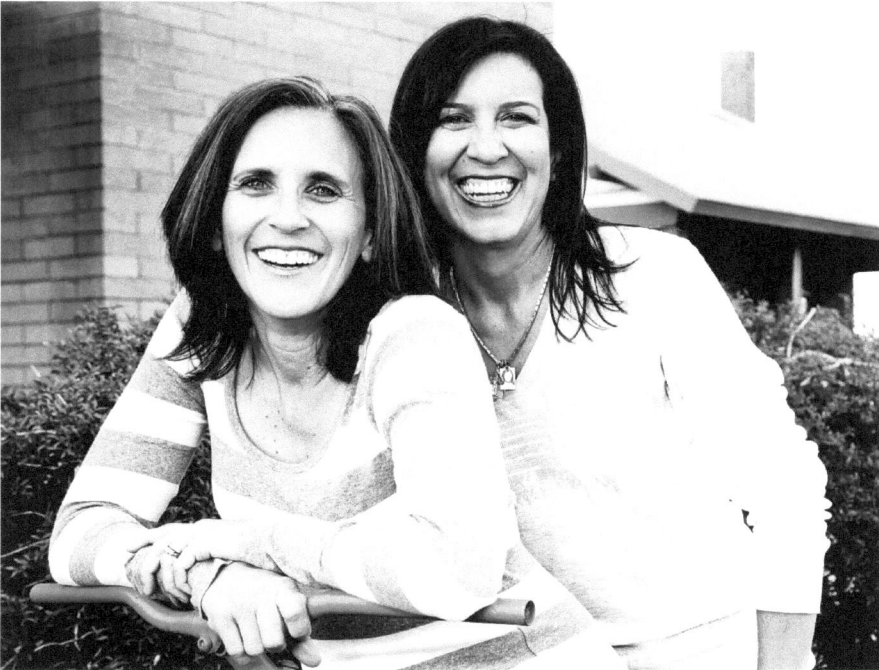

Epilogue

I count it a blessing to have been given the privilege to go to medical school in the United States. I got my M.D. in 1993 and thought I had reached the pinnacle of my career. So much time and energy invested in getting to that point. Then there was internship, then residency and finally GI fellowship. Along the journey, there were many exciting side trips such as being stationed in Guam with the Navy where I got to practice as an Internist at the Naval Hospital. From there I went back to training to become a Gastroenterologist.

Again, I want to be clear that I am ever so grateful for the honor of becoming a physician, I am so grateful to all the teachers and mentors I have had along the way. I say this, because what I am about to say is in no way a slam to anyone who has taught or mentored me. In fact, I would not even be here if it were not for all these wonderful teachers/mentors I have had. But, the reality is that after ten years of medical training no one really taught us anything about the role nutrition plays in our digestive health.

For years now, I have seen thousands of patients who come in for a variety of different gastrointestinal (GI) issues. I perform colonoscopies, upper endoscopies, run labs, do ultrasounds, CAT scans, MRI's, sometimes repeating some of these tests, prescribe great drugs and still the patients come back with symptoms. Now, I realize there is always the issue of patient compliance (meaning are patients really doing what I ask them to do), but let's assume for now that the patients have been fully compliant with my recommendations. Why then do they continue to come back with symptoms?

A few years ago, I really started thinking heavily about the role of nutrition. As I asked patients about what they ate and drank, many would almost get defensive saying they have a good diet and that is not the problem. A few would admit that they did not have the greatest diet. Even in those who claimed to have a great diet, as I questioned them more it became evident that a good diet wasn't necessarily a healthy diet.

Unfortunately, it has been very difficult to really engage in a good discussion about nutrition in the office, because of time constraints. Due to reimbursement cuts by health insurance companies, we have been forced to see more patients on any given day, in order to be able to survive as a business. It is hard enough to address the ongoing symptoms and make a treatment plan in the small amount of time in the office, now throw in trying to do nutritional counseling. It just does not happen.

The fact of the matter is the Standard American Diet (SAD) has poisoned our bodies. The food we eat makes our bodies sick. The food we eat makes our bodies fat. The food we have grown up eating here in North America does not nurture us. The food is so devitalized that it cannot nourish our cells. The body can only put up with this for so long before it starts to deteriorate. Why is it that there is so much cancer, heart disease, stroke, diabetes, fatty liver, obesity, among other diseases in our country? How is it that these illnesses have increased over the past few decades, instead of decreasing with our ever advancing medical technology and pharmaceuticals?

I truly believe as we have become more medically advanced and now have the most amazing drugs available to treat almost anything, we feel we can eat or do anything we want and all we have to do is take a pill to solve all of our problems. In order to keep up with this fast paced life that we have created for ourselves, the food industry has created pre-packaged food to eat on the run, that if need be could sit on a shelf indefinitely with all the preservatives and chemicals it contains. We have a fast food restaurant on every corner to help make our lives easier. If that was not enough, just to give us that extra boost in the morning, we can pick up a sugar or artificial sugar loaded fancy coffee drink loaded with caffeine. We now eat for convenience instead of for purpose and as a result, our health, especially our digestive health, suffers.

I see young people in their 20's and 30's who have already been diagnosed with irritable bowel syndrome, fibromyalgia, chronic fatigue syndrome, and cancer. I do colonoscopies on young people in whom I find precancerous polyps. If they had waited until the age of 50 to have their first baseline screening colonoscopy, there is a good chance they would not have even made it to that age because those precancerous polyps would have turned into colon cancer. This is what has happened to our fast pace, rushed, technologically advanced society. We are so advanced in so many areas and yet we neglect the things that are most important. It makes me sad.

I felt like I needed to find another answer. The drugs I was prescribing should have been helping my patients, but even they were not cutting it. I started doing my own research. I needed to do something! My patients needed a different answer, something that actually worked. I read a ton of books, spoke with many industry experts and finally landed on what I believe is the answer. And after trying it out on myself, my family and patient after patient it seems to be working.

The answer is not a fancy fad diet; there are no shots, no pills, no calorie counting, and no frills. If you want to feel better, eliminate your digestive issues, get your energy back and maybe even lose weight, I have a very simple answer for you. It is not a diet but a way of life that anyone can take on immediately. I hope that the contents of this book will inspire you to take action. I hope it will inspire you to think twice about what you put in your mouth. I hope I will be able to paint a picture of digestive wellness that will inspire you to change your life forever.

Our story

"Doc I'm just not digesting well," this is something I hear day in and day out as a Gastroenterologist. I have been practicing Gastroenterology for over a decade now and it seems I am getting busier and busier with each passing year. From the time I started practicing medicine I have had a very strong desire to spend time with my patients – listening to them, examining them, and really trying to get to the root of their issues. Around 2007 when I started my own practice, I noticed my patient panel start to shift. I started seeing many more young people in their 20's and 30's with the same digestive issues I was used to seeing in 50 and 60 year olds (including having precancerous polyps). I was running tests and doing procedures on all ages only to find nothing medically wrong which made treating the patients symptoms difficult. I was telling more and more patients they were going to have to be on prescription or non-prescription drugs indefinitely. This does not sit well with most, especially the younger patients.

My staff will tell you that I am the type of doctor that truly cares about my patients' well-being. When the answer is not there, Dr. Cruz will find it. But I have to admit, what was happening with the patients in my practice was stumping me time and time again. One day I approached my Office Manager, Tina Nunziato, who is also my life partner, and I asked her what we could do for these patients that were having digestive symptoms with no known cause. Her response was, "I don't know, but let's find out." That led us on a three year journey to discovering some pretty interesting facts about three key industries – food, healthcare and pharmaceuticals. After reading a ton of books, going to seminars, and talking with industry experts, I realized very quickly how little my medical degree actually taught me about nutrition and digestion.

Please know that I feel honored and privileged to have gone to medical school but knowing what I know now I feel sad that our medical schools are so focused on teaching us to find the symptoms and treat with drugs or surgery instead of really trying to get to the root cause. On average my patients are on 12 – 15 medications and we think this is how medicine should be. Unfortunately we are not healing patients like this; we are merely putting band-aids on very simple issues. In addition, by treating patients with this methodology, we are causing bigger issues and even more symptoms. Most of my patients cannot even remember what it feels like to be well. The question is, when will it end? When will patients realize enough is enough, and actually want to feel better again? Tina and I felt it was our mission to teach our patients what we learned so they could make more educated decisions for themselves when it comes to their health and their body.

Tina and I started incorporating our learning into our own life and the lives of our children. We felt if we were going to promote a better way of living we better be models to others. We started to shift what we ate, what we drank, what supplements we took, how we approached stress, etc. Although it took us a full two years to transition our lives I cannot even begin to explain what it has done for us as individuals and as a family. We are now healthier than ever, no more aches and pains, no more foggy brain, no more trips to the doctor, no more time off school and work. We have more energy than ever; the kids are strong and well developed both physically and mentally and we all continue to desire healthy food and drink.

In order to help me deliver our message to patients, Tina went back to school for her Holistic Nutrition Certificate. She helped me to craft and deliver our 12 week wellness program to any patient that was willing to listen and learn. Within 2 years we had helped dozens of patients improve and / or eliminate their digestive issues, get off some or all of their medications, regain their energy levels and in some cases even lose a considerable amount of weight. We noticed that as we taught, patients would grasp for more, and the more they grasped, the more we offered. We began partnering with service providers to offer colon hydrotherapy, infrared sauna treatments, lymphatic massage, etc. We partnered with dozens of vendors to provide healthy food and water to our patients at a discounted cost. It seemed like everyone who was introduced to the concepts we were teaching found a golden nugget that changed their life. The most interesting was the golden nugget was different for everyone.

As many of you know, with every great accomplishment comes an even bigger challenge. We were having a hard time keeping up with all the people we helped – we realized how difficult only having two educators can be. We noticed that if the patients did not have someone encouraging them or making them accountable they were having a hard time staying on track, no matter how bad they wanted good health. We have learned firsthand that it is very difficult to break years or even decades of unhealthy habits – whether it pertains to eating, drinking or stress. Without constant support and guidance it makes living a healthier life very difficult. We were spending so much time on the upfront education we weren't able to be there for everyone on the back-end to help them keep up the good work. In addition, due to constant reimbursement cuts year after year from the insurance companies I was being forced to see more patients in the office during the day which was making it more difficult to present our concepts to patients in the exam room.

This was a very difficult time for us and there were many times we wanted to quit. Although we were helping people we felt like we were not making the lifelong impact we were hoping for. In addition, we were not able to reach as many as we were before and it just seemed like we could not talk fast enough to enough people. No matter how frustrating it was at times, Tina and I both felt God continuing to push us forward in our mission. When we finally came to terms that quitting was not an option we realized we had to put some major thought into what we were doing and how we were doing it. We needed to come up with a way to deliver our products and services to take "US" out of the equation so we could spend our whole time supporting and guiding. This thought process took us almost a year. After attending a couple business seminars we crafted a delivery model that allows us to make the biggest impact and change the most lives for good.

We decided to package our teaching into a comprehensive 3 step program called the *"DNA for Digestive Health."* We knew we had a lot to share with people and we did not want to leave anything out; however we wanted to make it as simple as possible. The D stands for Detoxification and Digestive Restoration. The N stands for Nutrition and Necessary Hydration and the A stands for Activating the Mind, Body and Soul and Action Plan. All of which are crucial to changing a persons' digestive health. Aside from the fact that the acronym works well with the concepts we teach, the *"DNA for Digestive Health,"* is the structure one needs to follow to experience lasting results. What we have found personally is that once you begin on your path to digestive wellness it is almost like the DNA in your body actually does start to change. You begin craving the right foods and being disgusted by the wrong foods. You literally will be able to connect with your body again and feel when something is or is not good for it. You will feel amazing. It is really difficult to describe unless you have experienced it for yourself. It is like trying to explain what a rose smells like when the person has never been exposed to the scent of a flower.

Once you have created your *"DNA for Digestive Health"* plan we invite you to participate in our online community called "**www.DigestiveRevolution.com.**" This is where Tina and I spend most of our time adding resources, supporting and guiding those that desire life-long health. By delivering our key teachings online through home study materials, webinars, tele-seminars, and videos it will allow you to access the materials each day when it is most convenient for you. It will also free us up so we can spend more time guiding and supporting on a regular basis, which will help you stay on track with your digestive health goals and not feel like you are in it alone. None of us are perfect and it is going to be very important to have a community of supporters to help you get back on the bandwagon when you fall off.

Who is this book for?

This book is especially for each and every one of my patients or any person out there in need of a gastroenterologist because they have had or continue to have digestive issues. Digestive issues include but are not limited to:

- Constipation
- Diarrhea
- Bloating
- Gas
- Stomach Pain
- Acid Reflux / GERD
- Hemorrhoids
- Anemia
- Colitis
- Diverticulitis
- Crohn's
- Barrett's Esophagus
- Fatty Liver / High Liver Enzymes
- Irritable Bowel – IBS / IBD
- Pacreatitis
- Gallbladder issues

Those of you with digestive issues are not the only ones that can benefit from these teachings. Individuals with the following illnesses have also improved considerably after learning from us:

- Diabetes
- Heart Disease
- High Blood Pressure
- High Cholesterol
- Arthritis
- Allergies
- Cancer
- ADHD
- Autism
- Fibromyalgia

This book is also for those of you beginning to feel or have experienced for a long period of time the following symptoms which again, if not addressed will lead to more problematic symptoms, disease, surgery and one medicine after another:

- Low Energy
- Sluggishness
- High Fatigue
- Brain Fog
- Aches and Pains
- Difficulty Sleeping / Sleep Apnea
- Depression
- High Stress
- Lack of Movement
- Weight Gain

Finally, for those of you that are health nuts and are always staying on top of the most recent health craze we believe you will find our concepts a breath of fresh air. No matter who you are, if you started reading this book because it caught your attention, it probably is for you.

I do want to add however that if you are suffering from digestive issues or any health issue for that matter, in addition to reading this book you absolutely must see your doctor. This book is not meant to be a substitute for the care of a physician, but rather lessen the frequency for one over the long term. I always tell my patients before I teach them anything about digestive health and wellness that I want to make sure there is nothing medically wrong that we need to be aware of. After that I say, let the learning begin!

Outcome of our teachings

We are proud to say that everyone that has implemented what we are teaching has found something that works for them. They were able to find one thing that actually healed them or got to the bottom of the problem they were having. These problems could have been something that just started happening or problems they had for months if not years. The main outcome of our teachings is to try all the strategies to identify the one if not two concepts that answer the question, how can I feel better again without drugs and or surgery.

Our goal has always been to help you eliminate your digestive issues forever to reduce time with doctors, time off work, and money spent on tests, drugs and procedures. We also try to help as many of you as we can get off some or all of your medications. We try to show you how to turn your spending on illness into investing in your health. The reality is getting sick is a whole lot more expensive than staying healthy. By investing a little now in creating a healthy digestive system, you will save yourself thousands, maybe even tens of thousands of dollars over the course of your life. You are going to spend the money one way or the other. I do not know about you but I would much rather spend it on being healthy.

The effect of putting these principals into action has been amazing. When our patients' symptoms started going away almost everyone felt more energy, less fatigue and some even lost weight. It is not our goal from the beginning to make what we teach all about weight loss. We know weight loss is the hot topic – it has and always will be. The more important issue by far should be your health. There is no point in hitting your goal weight if you are unhealthy and feel sick all the time. Weight loss comes with a healthy body and it is usually the last thing that comes. Those people that stick with what we are teaching have the best results when it comes to weight loss. Not only do they hit their goal weight but many of their medical issues have improved and in some cases resolved.

Another major outcome of our teaching is changing the taste buds of the body and actually getting you to crave the food and drink the body needs instead of what the brain is telling you it wants. There are many big misconceptions about food and the body and we try to explain each one in detail to help move you toward the necessary transformation your body desires. Our bodies heal naturally, all we have to do is get out of the way.

Finally, we have found that our teachings will help you become the authority on digestive health. Many that have incorporated our teachings in their own lives have gone on to inspire friends and family members to do the same. Feeling good and looking good is contagious. When people around you realize that it is not normal for everyone to be feeling tired, on medications, and gaining weight they start to wonder how they can feel good too. Time and time again we have had people tell us they thought it was normal to feel tired all the time, have low energy, have symptoms, be on medications, gain weight, etc. because they were getting older and all of their friends were experiencing the same things. Let me be the first to tell you, you do not have to live your life like that. There is an answer and the answer is amazingly simple and so delicious!

How this book will benefit you

Before you even make the commitment to truly getting well and getting rid of your digestive issues for good you have to understand how the body works and why it is so important to embark on this mission. This book is going to teach you just that! Without this up front knowledge you will falter and you probably will fail because there is no background explaining the why. The why we have found is the most important thing for you to understand in order to be successful in anything.

By the time you finish reading this book you will have a better understanding of how your digestive system works, what is important to the body, what has been and continues to damage the body and how to begin turning the body around with a few very simple concepts. Let me also add that it is never too late to turn the body around. We have people in their 80's and 90's who are incorporating our teachings into their lives and seeing marked improvement in how they feel.

Our goal for this book is to teach you what you need to know to make the best decision for you going forward. Do you want change? Do you want to truly get rid of your digestive issues? If you do we are going to show you how. No time is better than the present to start the transformation that will change your life forever.

Structure and function of the body

"Doc, I'm not changing my diet and I'm not going stop drinking until the day I have cancer."

I have pleaded with this patient visit after visit to change his diet, stop drinking alcohol or at least cut back. He feels it needs to be a daily occurrence. He had prostate cancer six years ago, is obese, has a fatty liver and was recently found to have a spot on his liver. He was given a warning sign with the prostate cancer six years ago, but it has not hit home. This is not unusual. The bond we have with food and drink is an emotional one to the point of not being rational. We let our emotions drive how and what we eat and drink. We don't think with our brains to decide if it is good for us. Will it nourish our cells? Will it nourish our body?

To truly understand disease and symptoms of disease you need to learn a few basic biology principals about how your body works. This will help you understand that what is happening on the inside is affecting how you feel or look on the outside. The first lesson is about the structure and function of the body.

Our body is composed of trillions of cells that are continually repairing and renewing every minute of every day. There are thousands of specialized cell types, such as bone cells, skin cells, blood cells, nerve cells, brain cells, and so forth. Each cell type possesses a very specific structure, shape, function, and chemical make-up. It is this unique chemical make-up that gives each cell its properties. For cells to remain healthy and function perfectly as intended, and reproduce accurately they must be nourished by our blood. The blood carries the necessary building blocks out to the cells.

The building blocks that build a human cell include food, water and oxygen. When your diet is missing or lacking nutrients, you are denying cells what they need to function or live. If your cells lack nutrients long enough, they become weak and die. This causes toxic buildup and leads to your body breaking down from the inside out. Some bodies more than others.

Now that you know our health is dependent on healthy food, water and oxygen, there are really only two ways you can get sick, feel sluggish or have any health symptom whatsoever. The first way is when you are exposed to germs that your body cannot fight off. The second way is your body develops deformed or sick cells in weak areas causing such things as digestive issues, cancer, heart disease, diabetes, etc. In both cases, the causes are the same: your immune system is weakened, your cells are not functioning as they should and toxins are wreaking havoc on your body. For this to happen, it all comes back to one or a combination of all three of the following causes:

- You have nutritional deficiencies
- You have too many toxins in your body
- You have trapped mental and emotional stress

Has your doctor ever mentioned any of this to you before? Probably not. Yet these are the top three things causing issues in an unhealthy body. Let us dive deeper now and understand how the structure and function of the body relates to how we digest food.

The process of digestion

On one of Tina's recent trips to the grocery store she was picking out some English cucumbers when a nice woman came up to her and said, "You know sweetie I pick those cucumbers over in that bin because they're cheaper." Tina thanked her, but it crossed her mind that she should tell her that she buys English cucumbers because the skin is easier to digest and we should always eat the skin of our cucumbers. If you watch shoppers in the produce section, you will find them gathered around the bin with the cheapest vegetables. Tina saw an older couple reviewing the prices of lettuce a few weeks ago. In the end they decided to get the iceberg lettuce because it was the cheapest. There was no thought to which lettuce was healthier.

The next thing we need to discuss is how your body processes the food you eat. I need to ask you to stick with me for the next few minutes. I promise to make this biology lesson a quick one, everything you need to know about the process of digestion in just a few easy to read pages. Again, it is really important to know the how to understand the why. As a Gastroenterologist, this is where my specialty lies, the digestive system.

The digestive system starts in the mouth and ends in the anus. As food or liquid enters your mouth it is broken down by the teeth and acid found in saliva. As you swallow the food passes through your esophagus into your stomach. Your stomach produces acids and enzymes to break down your food into a more liquid form. The liquefied food then enters and travels through about 20 - 22 feet of small intestine (small bowel) and ends in the colon. The colon is also called the large bowel / intestine, which itself is about 5 or 6 feet long. Whatever does not get absorbed in the body comes out as something we know as poop, also called stool or feces.

Just like the plumbing system of a house is designed to direct fresh water and wastewater where it needs to go, the digestive system is designed to direct food and liquid in a way that will hopefully provide nutrition to help our body to grow healthy cells, tissue, and organs. If you look at a picture of the digestive system (Figure 1), it is a very simple looking collection of organs; a hollow tube spanning 29 feet in length. What goes on in this hollow tube however is much more complex and complicated than it appears, so let me break it down for you.

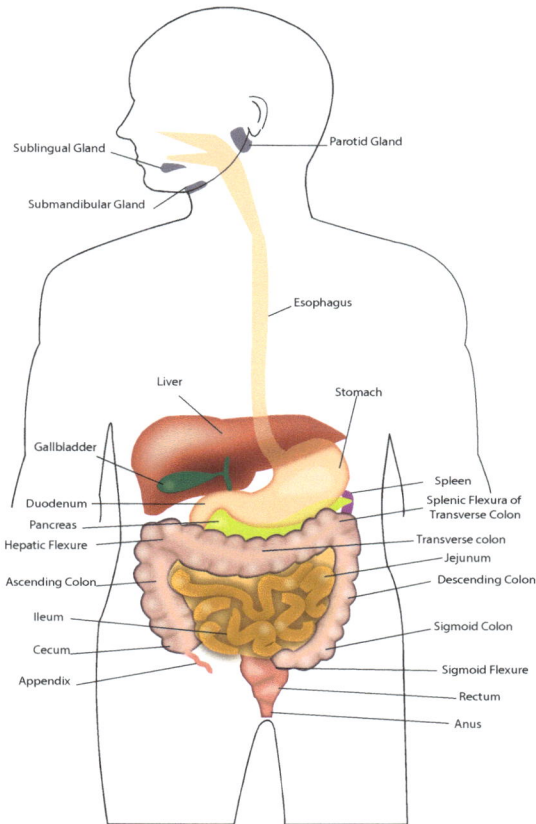

Figure 1

The food we eat has to be broken down and digested so we can absorb the nutrients which then feed our cells and body. The breakdown of food starts in the mouth with chewing. Chewing is one of the most important parts of the digestive process, because it makes it easier on the stomach to break down food. You have to remember that your stomach does not have teeth. If you are not thoroughly chewing your food, your body will not be able to break down your food properly to get the nutrients you need. A good rule of thumb is to chew each piece of food for at least 10 seconds.

Digestive enzymes start the chemical breakdown of food in the mouth. In fact, the moment you start to think about eating, the mouth starts to water. Contained in this liquid are the digestive enzymes getting ready to do their job.

As chewed food enters the stomach, gastric juices mix with the food to break it down into specific nutrients. Semi-liquid food called chyme enters the small intestine.

Additional digestion takes place in the beginning of the small intestine as more digestive juices from the pancreas and liver are dumped into the small intestine to help break down the nutrients. It is here in the small intestine where most of the absorption of nutrients takes place through little finger-like projections called villi (Figure 2). Absorption is the process where substances move through the wall of the intestine and enter the bloodstream. Villi protrude up from the small intestine. There are millions and millions of villi that allow for the absorption of nutrients that feed the cells throughout our body. If you were to

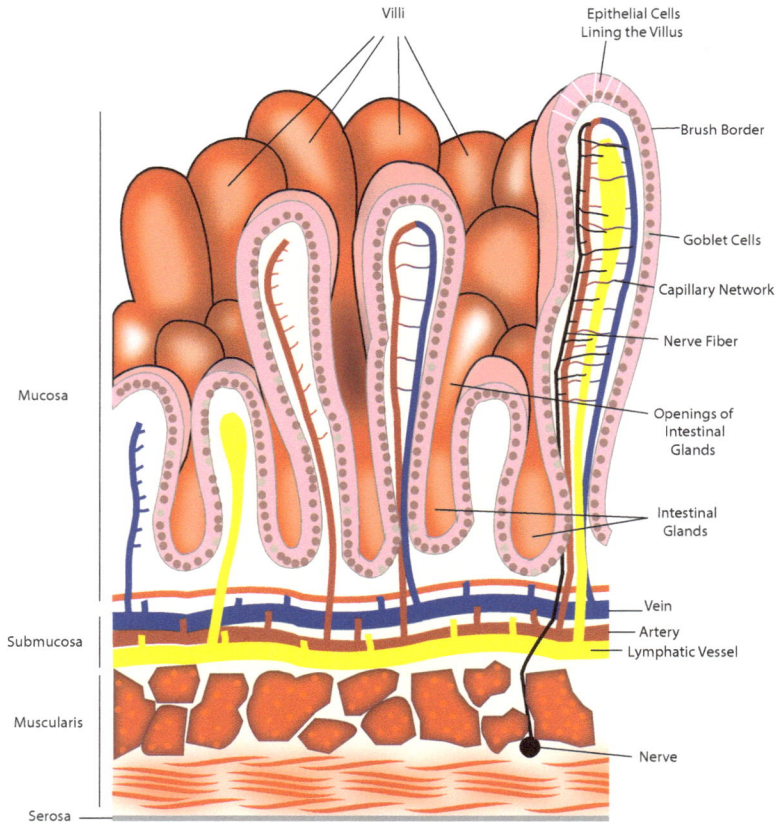

Figure 2

lay out all of these villi side-by-side it would cover the size of a football field.

Metabolism is the third stage of digestion and a series of chemical reactions conducted by individual cells in the body. These chemical reactions include breaking down food to harvest energy and building the parts that together make up cells. The nutrients taken by the blood will be processed by each cell to make every cell activity in the body happen. This is the process that gives life to our bodies.

By the time chyme reaches the large intestine (colon) most of the absorption of nutrients has taken place. In the colon is where stool or poop begins to form. Although there are no villi in the large intestine water, salts, vitamins and nutrients continue to be absorbed. Because there are no villi however, absorption is slower and not as efficient.

The colon is nothing but a large muscle and the goal of this muscle is to squeeze the chyme and with the help of bacteria undigested food is broken down to release even more nutrients into the bloodstream. The bacteria are responsible for the production of certain vitamins, including vitamin K and some B vitamins. It could take 1-3 days for material to pass through the colon. If it takes less time, you could get more liquid stools (diarrhea), if it takes it longer than 3 days, the stool could dry up making it very hard to come out, thus leading to constipation.

So there you have it, the digestive process from start to finish. Very simple and very cool – right? As you may know the colon is one of our major organs of elimination. Your next lesson is on the other five organs of elimination. If you do not understand how all the organs of elimination work together you will never understand the concept of toxicity – which is one of the main reasons we are all so sick and tired.

Organs of elimination

A client recently started our program and being an overachiever she thought she could incorporate all the teachings right away without creating a plan and easing into. We prepared her for the fact that although she could do this she needed to be aware that this tactic will cause her body to detoxify very quickly and could produce unpleasant side effects. As soon as she started she felt very sick. We told her the more toxic her body was the more severe her reaction would be as her body started cleaning out. There are two main points of the detoxification process, clearing out the toxins and rebuilding with food and water. Instead of deciding to take it a little slower she decided to quit because she did not like the way it made her feel. She went back to her fast food, junk food and multiple cups of coffee a day. It is not uncommon to experience what is called "a healing crisis" when going through detoxification, and although it may not feel good at the time, it is absolutely necessary to get back control of your body. If you start to feel aches and pains, headaches, flu like symptoms, etc. once you start to detoxify, don't give up! That just means it is working.

Did you know your colon is only one of many ways your body eliminates toxins or waste products? In order to get the whole picture you need to understand your organs of elimination and how toxins make their way out of your body.

Real healing is more than just the disappearance of symptoms. The body must eliminate toxins and waste products efficiently and completely or the system becomes overloaded and stressed. When not eliminated, waste products settle in the tissues and symptoms of ill health, including digestive issues, low energy, weight gain, and aches and pains, make their appearance.

The body has six organs of elimination:

- Bowel (Large Intestine)
- Lungs
- Skin
- Kidneys
- Liver
- Lymphatic System

The large bowel (also known as the large intestine / colon) eliminates waste, including unused food from the body. This organ is not made of metal or concrete to hold in all the toxic substances, it is made of tissue. Toxins from stagnating wastes in the bowel find their way into the bloodstream. This in turn means that the blood that circulates through the bowel also circulates through the brain. Many believe that a clean unobstructed bowel leads to a clear mind and a balanced body. People do not associate their headaches and sluggishness to slow transit of waste through the body. Most will be amazed how much better they feel once the organs of elimination are toned and regulated.

The lungs eliminate carbon dioxide and provide fresh oxygen for cells. The lungs also help to excrete harmful products we ingest, for instance overheated oil from fried foods through carbon dioxide elimination. Our cells require oxygen in order to carry out proper metabolism. Poor oxygen circulation results in a tired body and mind. One of the things we teach in our program is the importance of deep breathing. Most of us breathe shallow breaths a majority of the time causing less oxygen to enter our bloodstream which contributes to us feeling so tired all the time.

The skin receives one third of the body's circulating blood and should eliminate one third of the body's wastes through sweat and perspiration. It is important to allow the skin to perspire and sweat freely so this can happen. Avoid excessive soap, antiperspirants, and cosmetics which clog pores and prevent free elimination. Body odor and bad breath are important indicators of internal health. If you are healthy your body and breath should not be offensive. We noticed when we started eating healthier and putting less chemicals into our body that our sweat did not smell anymore. When we do splurge and eat something outside the realm of our normal diet within days our sweat smells again.

The liver aids in digestion and disperses the products of digestion into the bloodstream and the small intestine. The kidneys filter the products of digestion, cell metabolism, and liver detoxification from the blood. The kidneys are the end-stage filtering system of the body and are constantly filtering our blood. The products of digestion enter the kidneys and are excreted through urine. When the kidneys and liver are not functioning efficiently, waste products remain circulating in the blood and the body retains fluid. This results in a loss of appetite, weight gain, a general feeling of discomfort, tiredness, nausea, and even vomiting. If left unaddressed, this could eventually lead to the onset of disease.

The lymphatic system cleanses and protects the body from invading bacterial substances by preventing them from entering the bloodstream. This system is composed of lymph nodes and lymphatic vessels that are filled with lymph, a whitish, watery fluid (Figure 3). Unlike the blood, which has the heart to pump it, the lymphatic system does not have its own circulatory pump. It relies on the movement of the muscles to move the lymph fluid around the body. If the lymph nodes become congested with toxins, they cannot properly perform their task. Symptoms of a clogged lymphatic system are recurring throat and tonsil problems, swollen glands (enlarged lymph nodes), and sometimes tumors. Our lymph system runs throughout our whole body. A large amount of drainage is near the breasts in women and near the groin in men. Many believe breast and prostate cancer are so prevalent because of clogged lymphatic systems.

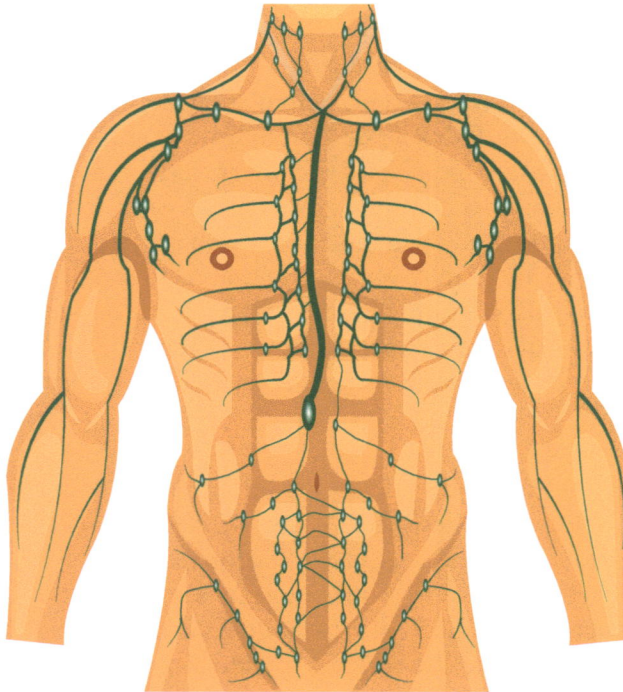

Figure 3

Many people will blame their ill health or symptoms on the fact that they are genetically predisposed to certain diseases. They will say things like, "my Dad had high blood pressure so that is why I have it." Or, "my Mother had cancer so I am bound to have cancer." What you should know is, genetics play a minor role in the outcome of our health.

The food we put in our mouths and how it is digested, assimilated, metabolized and eliminated is a major factor. How we choose to take care of our body, plays a major role in the outcome of our health.

If our food choices are not good we are not nourishing our bodies or eliminating properly. I am sure many of you believe you eat a healthy well-balanced diet. Let me say that if you are shopping in standard grocery stores, eating out regularly and eating what is considered the Standard American Diet you are definitely not eating a well balanced diet. I know this to be true because we felt we were eating healthy, that is until we learned what we know now. Do not kid yourself; the digestive issues you are dealing with have a direct correlation to what you are eating.

Why digestive issues are not your fault

How did we get so sick, fat, tired and dependent on drugs and sugar?

How do you feel these days? Run down, exhausted, brain fog, aches and pains, low energy, digestive problems, unexplained weight gain? Don't worry it's not just you. Nine times out of ten the patients we deal with every day have these exact same issues. Look around you, at your family, your friends, your coworkers. Everyone seems to be sick, fat, tired and / or dependent on drugs and sugar. So how did this happen? We don't remember it ever being as bad as it is today and it does not seem like it is going to get any better. In fact it seems like it is only getting worse with each passing year.

In the grand scheme of things there are only a few things that are truly affecting why we are so sick, fat, tired and dependent on drugs and sugar:

- The healthcare / pharmaceutical industry – our medical system is setup to diagnose and treat disease with procedures, surgeries and drugs. Medicine is about treating diseases not preventing them.
- The food industry – our nation is consistently consuming food and drink that is difficult to digest and offers little to no nourishment to the body. The Standard American Diet (SAD) is sad for a reason. We are an over fed, under nourished, toxic and dehydrated society.
- Our high stress lifestyle – every single person we work with is stressed out about something, whether it is money, relationships, work, or family. High levels of stress lead to major health problems and a lack of sleep which in and of itself is unhealthy.
- Our stagnate society – most of us spend a majority of our day in a chair, in front of a computer, watching television or in the case of our children playing video games. We are too busy being entertained to get out and move our bodies and be active.

The next section of this book will go into detail on these four areas and how these things have caused us to be so sick, fat, tired and dependent on drugs and sugar. Here is why you are not totally to blame and how to work around these issues to get yourself back to good health.

The problem with healthcare and pharmaceuticals

The medication lists that patients bring in to their appointments these days are amazingly long. It is not unusual to see 5-10 medications, but I'm seeing longer lists these days. I have patients with 20 or more medications on their lists. Some of these patients are young. I am particularly saddened when I see patients who can barely stay awake at their appointments because of the narcotics they are taking. Young patients admit to me they cannot live without their narcotics. I recently saw a young woman who came in with a diagnosis of irritable bowel syndrome, gastroesophageal reflux disease, arthritis, and fibromyalgia. She had just had a complete hysterectomy for endometriosis and came in on a long list of medications including narcotics. Her arms were covered with pain medication patches. I just wanted to cry when I saw this young girl. What are we doing to this girl? She should not have all these diagnoses. She is too young. Her mother pleaded with me to please save her daughter. No one else in the family had any medical problems.

Remember back in the day when a physician would actually come to your house when you were sick? Well, as we know, those days are long gone. So many chronic health issues developed that the industry of medicine had to compartmentalize. In 1950, the concept of sub-specialists was created. Multiple physicians were now caring for us instead of just one. When this transition happened in medicine it was not about treating the whole person anymore, it was about treating an organ or set of organs in the body.

In medical school physicians learn how the body works, how to diagnose a disease and how to treat the disease with surgery or drugs. There is hardly any training on nutrition or how what we eat affects our bodies. In medicine, reimbursements are made based on number of visits, surgeries or procedures performed and drugs administered. It has nothing to do with preventing disease. When entering medical school, students must take the Hippocratic Oath. It is widely believed to have been written by Hippocrates himself, the same philosopher who also wrote "let food be thy medicine…". The oath is a promise to practice medicine ethically and do no harm.

In more detail it means that a physician must abide by a certain standard of care called evidence based medicine. This type of medicine is based on trying to compile the best evidence out there so the healthcare system can formulate the best practices, protocols and treatments. Most of these studies are performed in all areas of drugs and surgery but rarely is there sufficient funding to study natural or holistic treatments. This is why many physicians are scared to practice preventive medicine or even consider that food could be the cause of disease.

To further the challenges in healthcare, in 1988, managed care HMO's were developed to contain rising medical costs. By 1995, the practice of medicine was affected by this new structure. The work of a physician became more about the numbers than patient care and physicians were forced to see more patients in less time. In the 21st century we have seen health insurance rates climb and physician reimbursements decline year after year. Physicians cannot afford to run their practices anymore and are shutting their doors. Fewer and fewer people want to become physicians. Wait times to see physicians are getting longer and longer, with many patients waiting months for an appointment.

When we get sick we go see our physicians. After waiting weeks or months to be seen, we might spend a total of 10 minutes with them, and we are lucky if they even touch or examine us. Because they have been taught to diagnose and treat, most of the time they will prescribe a medication and send us on our way. Even if we ask them what could be causing our symptoms many will admit they have no idea. Remember, this is not their fault; they were never trained to focus on prevention. How did this happen you ask? That leads us to the pharmaceutical industry.

There has been increasing controversy surrounding pharmaceutical companies and their influence on healthcare. In the early 1970's the pharmaceutical industry began to expand at a greater rate as the government allowed companies to own patents on drugs and the way drugs were manufactured. In 1975, pharmaceutical companies began investing in medical schools and nursing programs in turn influencing the curriculum. They sponsored events and placed ads in journals and at medical conferences. The use of prescription drugs grew dramatically.

In the mid 1980's pharmaceutical manufacturing was done by a few large companies that held a dominant position throughout the world. In 1997 direct-to-consumer advertising proliferated on radio and TV because of new FDA regulations that made it easy to present risks to drug consumers. Thousands of pharmaceutical lobbyists are in Washington D.C. lobbying Congress to protect their interests. Who is in Washington D.C. looking out for our interests?

On a separate note, safety studies managed by pharmaceutical companies have been in question for some time. Studies sponsored by pharmaceutical companies are several times more likely to report positive results, especially if a drug company employee is involved (as is often the case). There is a drug that has been created for every symptom out there. We have been trained as patients to ask for the drug instead of ask why a symptom exists so it can actually be fixed instead of just covered up with a pill.

Most drugs are not tested against other drugs to see if they create reactions or additional symptoms. On average people are taking 6-8 pharmaceutical drugs at the same time (with some taking 20 medications at the same time). We do not understand how these drugs are interacting in our bodies. One drug leads to another as side effects are inevitable. We continue to receive one drug after another to cover up our symptoms instead of trying to figure out how to solve the problem.

Why is it the more medicine we take, the worse we feel? We all know there is a time and place for prescription medication, like taking antibiotics for serious infections. If you find yourself taking drugs over a long period of time something is probably not right. Our bodies were designed to heal themselves (think about what happens when you get a cut). Is it possible for our self-healing bodies to really be that sick? We think not!

The problem with the food industry

Ever wonder where the food pyramid that we use as our nutritional Bible came from? You might remember the Four Basic Food Groups, an outdated concept that was conceived in the 1950's. The milk industry was happy since milk, eggs and cheese were one of the groups. The Improved American Food Guide Pyramid was adopted from Denmark by the USDA in 1992. Over the last few years the USDA modified that food pyramid to create one of their very own. The interesting thing about the food pyramid is that over the years there has been so much squabbling between the dairy and meat industry along with the medical and health organizations in regards to these food guidelines. You have to wonder if these guidelines are really meant to help us eat better or if they promote the sale of specific food items.

In 1977 the government spent quite a bit of time and energy trying to determine the cause of heart disease, cancer and diabetes in our nation. What they found was that the increase in these chronic diseases was directly linked to our diet. The Senate Select Committee on Nutrition held hearings on the topic and prepared a document that was to guide our nation to better health. What they found was this:

- Although rates of chronic disease soared in America since WWII, other countries consuming traditional diets based largely on plants had low rates of the same chronic diseases.
- During WWII when meat and dairy products were highly rationed, the rate of chronic disease in America temporarily plummeted.

Based on these findings, the Committee suggested a set of guidelines calling on Americans to cut down on red meat and dairy consumption. This, as you might guess, greatly upset the red meat and dairy industries. They attacked the Committee and demanded a rewrite. The guidelines were altered from "reduce consumption" to "choose meats, poultry and fish that will reduce saturated-fat intake". In addition, the beef lobbyists made sure the Senator that headed up the Committee was ousted during the next election. This sent a message to Washington that no one should be challenging the American diet, and no one has since.

From then on, the government avoided talk about whole foods, and instead spoke in scientific terms about nutrients, topics that most Americans did not understand. In 1982, the National Academy of Sciences issued a report on diet and cancer which did not criticize any specific food group. The report created new dietary language and the food industry and the media quickly followed suit. Terms like polyunsaturated, cholesterol, monounsaturated, carbohydrate, fiber, polyphenols, amino acids and carotenes soon described what was traditionally known as food. There was a promise of scientific certainty that if you ate more of the right nutrients and less of the wrong, you would live longer and avoid chronic disease. Ironically no one could decipher what right from wrong was.

This change in how we dialogued about food was deemed The Age of Nutritionism, where the key to understanding food was understanding its nutritional make-up. Because you cannot see a nutrient it made them seem extremely mysterious. So it fell on the scientists and journalists to explain the hidden reality of food to us. This new way of looking at food made it difficult to distinguish between foods. For example fish, beef and chicken through the scientist's eyes became different ways to ingest quantities of fats and proteins. This in turn, made it difficult to identify the differences between processed foods and whole foods, since the focus was on quantifying the nutrients they contained.

It was a great time for the manufacturers of processed foods. In 1982, the food industry began to reengineer thousands of popular food products to contain more of the nutrients that science and government had deemed to be good. By the late 1980's the era of food science was upon us. Real food likes fruits and vegetables had a hard time competing. You cannot change the chemical balance of an avocado or put oat bran in an apple. It was a lot easier to put a health claim on a can or box than on a fruit or vegetable.

The National Academy of Sciences report also helped to encourage the low-fat diet craze. Food manufacturers began producing low-fat versions of many popular foods. Oddly, Americans kept getting fatter on this new low-fat diet. The current obesity and diabetes epidemic happened right around the same time that Americans began consuming more carbohydrates as a way to avoid the evils of fat. What we failed to realize during this time is that although we

From then on, the government avoided talk about whole foods, and instead spoke in scientific terms about nutrients, topics that most Americans did not understand. In 1982, the National Academy of Sciences issued a report on diet and cancer which did not criticize any specific food group. The report created new dietary language and the food industry and the media quickly followed suit. Terms like polyunsaturated, cholesterol, monounsaturated, carbohydrate, fiber, polyphenols, amino acids and carotenes soon described what was traditionally known as food. There was a promise of scientific certainty that if you ate more of the right nutrients and less of the wrong, you would live longer and avoid chronic disease. Ironically no one could decipher what right from wrong was.

This change in how we dialogued about food was deemed The Age of Nutritionism, where the key to understanding food was understanding its nutritional make-up. Because you cannot see a nutrient it made them seem extremely mysterious. So it fell on the scientists and journalists to explain the hidden reality of food to us. This new way of looking at food made it difficult to distinguish between foods. For example fish, beef and chicken through the scientist's eyes became different ways to ingest quantities of fats and proteins. This in turn, made it difficult to identify the differences between processed foods and whole foods, since the focus was on quantifying the nutrients they contained.

It was a great time for the manufacturers of processed foods. In 1982, the food industry began to reengineer thousands of popular food products to contain more of the nutrients that science and government had deemed to be good. By the late 1980's the era of food science was upon us. Real food likes fruits and vegetables had a hard time competing. You cannot change the chemical balance of an avocado or put oat bran in an apple. It was a lot easier to put a health claim on a can or box than on a fruit or vegetable.

The National Academy of Sciences report also helped to encourage the low-fat diet craze. Food manufacturers began producing low-fat versions of many popular foods. Oddly, Americans kept getting fatter on this new low-fat diet. The current obesity and diabetes epidemic happened right around the same time that Americans began consuming more carbohydrates as a way to avoid the evils of fat. What we failed to realize during this time is that although we did eat more carbohydrates to avoid fats, we really did not eat less fat. Meat consumption actually rose during this time. So we had just added more carbohydrates to our plate to cover up the ever increasingly large piece of meat.

When too many carbohydrates became the focus of why everyone was getting fatter, Atkins mania hit the food industry and breads and pastas were given a quick redesign (pulling back the carbohydrates and increasing the protein). The message during this time basically gave us permission to eat MORE low-fat food and we did just that. In addition, we continued to educate ourselves about food from the outside package and we believed every claim, true or not. Why would food companies lie to us? We were being protected by our government right?

We are provided food with little nutrition from cradle to grave and wonder why we do not feel good by the time we hit our mid 20's. We want to chalk it up to getting old, but getting old has nothing to do with it. It just takes that long before our body starts reacting to the food we have been eating since birth. Have you ever looked at the ingredients of baby formula? You will be surprised to know that sugar and high-fructose corn syrup are among the leading ingredients.

We have become addicted to sugar at birth. If you think tobacco is hard to quit, try sugar. We love it, we cannot get enough of it, and the food manufacturers know it. They make it faster, cheaper, and easier and it lasts forever on the shelf. This is what we have told them is important to us. It is not about the quality of the food we put in our mouth it is about the best value for our money. Burgers off the dollar menu will always be cheaper than a head of broccoli at the grocery store, but what will those burgers cost you later? The answer is a lifetime of prescription medication, doctor's visits, hospital stays, medical procedures and surgeries. So what is actually the better value?

The food industry has done an amazing job at re-engineering what was food. It has been processed so much and contains so many chemicals that there are no nutrients left. Unbeknownst to us, we are filling our bodies with toxic chemicals and robbing them of nutrients causing us to get sick, fat and tired.

Toxicity = acidity, acidity = health problems

One of my patients is in her late 20's and her body is already beginning to shut down. She is overweight and had to have her gallbladder removed a couple years ago after having gallbladder attacks during pregnancy. Now, she is having kidney problems, headaches, body aches, and recurring colds that require her to take time off of work at least once a month. She admits she has no control over her eating habits. She eats fast food for breakfast, fast food for lunch and has some type of sweet treat every day. She eats very few vegetables and she admits she could go forever without drinking water. She only drinks soda, juice, tea, and coffee. No water whatsoever! No wonder the organs are shutting down one at a time. Fortunately, she's not in multi-organ failure requiring hospitalization. She has a chance. I told her these are her warning signs and she needs to listen. It is not rocket science. We do not need scientific studies here to know her body is starving for water and nutrition. This is not an unusual American story. I see this in my practice every day. We are starving our bodies. We are feeding our body nutritionally depleted food and drink and expect our body to keep us healthy!

How do we reverse the damage of years of toxic build up? It has to do with a theory that has been around for ages…

In medical school we learned about acid-base balance as it relates to a patient's illness mainly when they are hospitalized. We know that unless the body's pH is slightly alkaline, the body cannot heal itself. What is pH you ask? It stands for potential of Hydrogen. It is a value that indicates how acidic or alkaline a solution is. The higher the pH reading, the more alkaline or oxygen rich a solution. The lower the reading, the more toxic, acidic or oxygen-deprived a solution. pH values range from 0-14. The middle value of 7.0 is a neutral state. So any value greater than 7.0 is alkaline and any value less than 7.0 is acidic.

Human blood is slightly alkaline with a pH of 7.36-7.38. In fact if the pH of your blood goes to 7.1 or 7.7 you will die instantly. It is similar to holding your breath for more than 2 to 3 minutes. In medical school, internship, residency or even my gastroenterology training I do not ever recall any discussion or teachings, about how our diet can impact on our body's acid-base balance.

I certainly don't recall any teaching about how this acid-base balance could impact on our everyday health except as it related to patients who were hospitalized and seriously ill. We know now that the pH of your body affects your entire state of health including your weight.

A diet rich in acid-producing foods such as animal products, sugar, coffee, soda, and processed foods puts an enormous amount of pressure on the body to regulate its pH. As the body is trying to do this, it uses up its own supply of alkaline minerals such as potassium, magnesium, sodium, and calcium, making that person prone to chronic and degenerative diseases. Minerals are removed from bones and vital organs to help neutralize all the excess acid and remove it from the body.

Figure 4 shows a pH chart to give you a nice visual of this concept. We try to teach people to eat and drink higher than their blood pH (to the right of blood on the chart) to help their body out as much as possible.

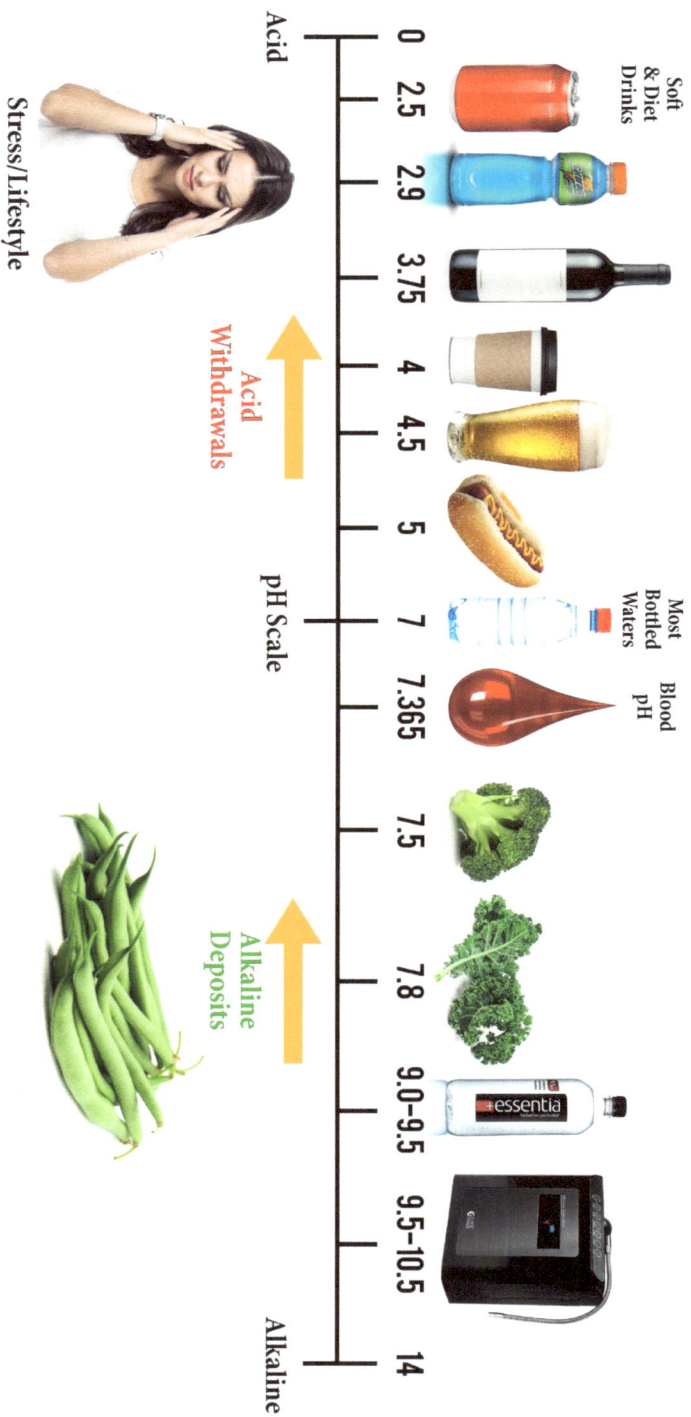

pH Chart

Acid

Stress/Lifestyle

pH Scale

0
2.5 — Soft & Diet Drinks
2.9
3.75
4 — Acid Withdrawals
4.5
5
7 — Most Bottled Waters
7.365 — Blood pH
7.5
7.8 — Alkaline Deposits
9.0-9.5 — +essentia
9.5-10.5
14

Alkaline

Figure 4

Research has shown unless the body's pH is normal (slightly alkaline) it cannot heal itself. It cannot effectively use vitamins, minerals and supplements. That is why someone who lives on junk food and fast food and feels it is okay because they take their daily multi-vitamin is only kidding themselves. High acid levels in their body (acidosis) make them unable to benefit from the multi-vitamin. In addition, maintaining an acidic environment in your body will promote and support the growth of microorganisms including bacteria, yeast, viruses, fungus, parasites and mold.

When your body fluids contain too much acid it is called acidosis. Proponents of the acid-alkaline theory believe that acidosis causes the following:

- Destroys the body's ability to absorb nutrients
- Decreases energy production in cells
- Decreases the body's ability to repair damaged cells
- Makes tumor cells thrive and grow
- Makes the body more prone to illness and fatigue
- Encourages the body to store fat to protect itself

I completely subscribe to this theory. It makes sense – look at how much disease is around us. We have the latest and greatest in medical technology yet there is more disease today than ever before. Is any of this sinking in?

The acid-alkaline concept focuses on the effect that food has on our body's pH level once the food is consumed. The body must maintain balance between two main types of chemicals: acids and alkalis. This balance creates what is called the pH value of our body's fluids. In order to function properly our cells require a slightly alkaline environment. The metabolic processes in our body are regularly producing acids. To keep healthy, the body is constantly trying to neutralize / buffer these acids and eliminate them. Once food is digested it will create an acidic effect or an alkaline effect in your body.

Good health or disease begins in the cells. In order for our cells to function properly, they need to receive life-giving nutrients and oxygen from the bloodstream and the cells also need to be able to release their waste. These functions occur optimally if the body is slightly alkaline. As the body becomes acidic the cell functions become impaired, there is decreased oxygen and nutrients being supplied to the cells and there is a build-up of waste in the cells. This sets the stage for fatigue, weight gain and disease – especially digestive disease.

Most likely everyone who has been eating the Standard American Diet for any length of time has high levels of acidosis. The body is an amazing creation that can bounce back from the effect of bad habits. Even if you have been in a chronic acidic state for years you can still derive great benefits, eliminate symptoms, lose weight and live much healthier if you help your body to regulate its pH. This concept has nothing to do with counting calories, fats, proteins, or carbohydrates. It simply has to do with eating less acidic foods and more alkaline foods. It is that simple.

How do you know which foods are more acidic and which foods are more alkaline? Tests have been conducted on many foods to identify their pH values. Most books on this topic will show varying results. We have taken all of these results and distilled them into a point system that we teach through our program. In general however, it is important to know that some foods by nature might seem acidic, such as tomatoes, lemons and limes, are actually very alkalizing once metabolized.

Another example is white bread, which by nature does not seem like an acidic food, but once it has been digested and metabolized the end product is actually very acidic. So the answers are not as simple as they might seem. In addition, it is important to know that there is an alkaline alternative to most acidic foods. For example pasta made from quinoa is more alkaline where pasta made from flour or wheat is more acidic. The key is knowing what the healthier alternatives are to everything you eat. Instead of saying you are not allowed to eat pasta anymore you just have to know which pasta to eat.

This is a very foreign concept for western world physicians and even dieticians and nutritionists who all want to focus on calories and the nutrients provided by foods. Certainly the nutritional value of food should not be ignored, but more important is how that particular food will affect the acid-alkaline balance in the body. The bottom line is that you want to keep the body in a slightly more alkaline state in order to optimize the environment for the cells to function properly. With a slightly more alkaline environment your body will be able to better absorb and use the nutrients that it needs from the food you have eaten.

The war against devitalized foods

A patient of ours drank two cans of Dr. Pepper and ate a package of Twinkies for breakfast every day without fail. She is a high powered executive, does a lot of traveling and came to us to see if we could help her with her weight gain, fatigue and lack of energy. She felt the lack of energy was due to her hectic travel schedule. Although this indeed could be a contributor to her fatigue and lack of energy, we suggested that her diet could be playing a part as well. She was quick to tell us that this was impossible as she had been eating this breakfast for years. She was willing to modify her hectic work and travel schedule, but made it clear she was not giving up her Dr. Pepper. She said it gave her a boost in the morning that she needed. We told her it would be difficult to help her until she realized what she was putting in her mouth was affecting the way she felt. We explained to her that Dr. Pepper and Twinkies are nutritionally depleted food and drink items. I think most people know this; they just don't want to admit it.

Devitalized food is food that has been stripped of nutrients, minerals, and vitamins during processing. Although devitalized foods sound terrible for our body, we are consuming more of them each day than anything else. Devitalized foods include:

- Fast food
- Sugar
- White flour
- White rice
- White pasta
- Table salt
- Processed foods- that come in cans, boxes or bags

We must start thinking about the food we eat as energy or fuel for the body. Each time you eat or drink you need to ask yourself, "is this going to give me life, healthy nutrients and vitality or is it going to take away life, nutrients and vitality?"

As Americans have gotten busier and busier over the last 30 years there has been a major shift in food consumption. We have stopped making wholesome food at home and instead eat in restaurants and on the run. Fast food not only includes drive through style fast food restaurants but also frozen microwavable meals. Did you know when we microwave foods we change the molecular composition of that food, stripping it of its nutrients? Have you ever put a piece of bread in the microwave? When you take it out and let it sit for a couple of minutes it gets as hard as a rock. Technically, it is not bread anymore.

Most fast food products have few if any nutrients and are bulked up with pasta, breadcrumbs, corn flour, processed potato, processed egg and milk products, hydrogenated vegetable oil, saturated fats, gums and sugar substitutes. They are given flavor by the addition of herbs and spices, salt, monosodium glutamate (MSG) and sugars. Fast food products also contain artificial colors, preservatives and artificial flavorings.

Far too many households eat a daily diet of microwavable ready meals with very little fresh foods included. Then they "treat" themselves to a meal out, by visiting a burger or pizza restaurant, or think a healthy meal is a steak and fries. There are studies that have shown fast food is extremely addictive. The high levels of salt and sugar found in most fast food items cause the brain to seek them out. Fast food is one of the hardest things to give up in the beginning; however, to maintain your digestive health and regulate your weight - YOU MUST EVENTUALLY ELIMINATE FAST FOOD FROM YOUR DIET ALTOGETHER!! It does not matter how long this process takes, it should be your ultimate goal.

Fast food is popular because it is quick, convenient, and usually inexpensive. You can buy fast food just about anywhere that sells food and snacks: vending machines, drive-through restaurants and 24 hour convenience stores. For under $5.00 you can get a filling meal. Fast food is inexpensive because it is made with cheap ingredients. When you think about it, although fast food is inexpensive it is costing you so much health and vitality. Here are some tips to help you avoid fast food:

- Eat with purpose, not convenience. Do not wait until you are hungry to decide what you are going to eat. Each day put some thought into what you will eat the next day. What do you have planned? When, where and what will you eat? Prepare your meals and snacks ahead of time and take them with you.
- If you absolutely need to get something quick choose a healthy alternative, for example Paradise Bakery instead of McDonald's or Burger King. Make a conscious decision to wait to eat until you are near healthier food. You must decide that a little hunger is a small price to pay to avoid a bad decision that will take your life force away.

Stress? What stress? I don't stress

One of our patients who is very stressed out with just about everything in her life, called us angry one day saying she could no longer drink the 3 glasses of wine she was accustomed to drinking on a daily basis. She was half way through the program and her main drink had now become water. She was also eating healthier foods on a regular basis. She was feeling great and believed she had detoxified. She was angry because she could not tolerate her alcohol anymore. Her body was rejecting the alcohol she felt she needed to calm her stresses. She had given her body a taste of good, healthy liquid and food and now was having a hard time getting the alcohol down. We advised her to cut down to one glass of wine per day to merely pacify her need for wine. Even though at the end of the program she was drinking one glass of wine per day, she admitted to us that it was even hard for her to get that down. Her body was trying to tell her something, but she insisted on giving it something it was rejecting. We told her the next important step for her is finding healthier ways to handle her stress so she doesn't feel like she needs the wine at all.

When we look at what kind of lives our grandparents lived I think we can admit our lives have become so much easier on some levels and yet so much more complicated on others. It has never been so easy to stay connected with family and friends with cell phones, email and social media. Products are available to make life easier in the home and at work. We don't have to travel as much for work since many things can happen over the internet. There is so much information available at the click of a mouse that we never go long without knowing the answer to our most recent questions.

On the flip side, all of these conveniences allow us to do more in one day than our grandparents were able to do in a week. We cannot live without our cell phones, computers and other electronic devices. It is the norm for even young children to have cell phones and the latest handheld devices. We are hard on ourselves and hard on everyone around us and we set expectations that are often times unreachable. We live in a state of chronic stress.

We do not have enough time for our children, or our spouse, much less ourselves. We are driving ourselves to the grave. The incidence of depression and anxiety has never been higher. Over 25% of our patients are on some form of antidepressant or anti-anxiety drug. On top of that we do not exercise as we should. No wonder plastic surgeons and bariatric surgeons are busier than ever.

We are getting fatter and aging more quickly than ever before. Life is a merry-go-round and we cannot figure out how to get off.

So, how did we get here? What happened to the simple life? It seems we have gone and made it complicated. Because of the high expectations we have set, we have made ourselves and our children busier than ever. It is not enough to be involved in just one thing; we have got to do it all. We strive to keep up with the Jones' and have become more materialistic than ever. Never happy with what we have, we always need the next best thing. This may mean we are living above our means and have become reliant on credit cards. Being in debt is one of the top stressors for families these days.

Stress and anxiety can actually be a good thing to motivate us to take action. It becomes unhealthy when we are worried and anxious about things that are out of our control, things that have not happened yet, or when it paralyzes us to the point where we don't have the desire to take action anymore. Stress and anxiety are problems of the mind. We may have a very simple worry or concern that keeps torturing our mind to the point of pushing out all other thoughts.

This tower of worry tends to repeat itself over and over in our minds because stress and anxiety tend to recreate themselves. Our minds become conditioned to anxiety and worry to the point that it returns quickly to stress and anxiety as an automatic reflex. This causes a problem not only for our mind, but for our bodies.

It is amazing how the mind controls the body. We create a storm within our own minds that in most situations is only an illusion. This stress and anxiety causes physical symptoms and real medical problems including headaches, high blood pressure, ulcers, sleep problems, joint pain, lowered immune system, irritability, anger outbursts, bowel problems, difficulty with concentration, depression, memory problems, as well as problems with alcohol and drug abuse. This is when we must look inside to figure out what is causing us to worry.

So, what else does stress do to the body? It uses up energy. When the body burns energy, it creates acid. So we become more acidic and thus more toxic. We create negative energy. Being acidic and toxic makes us susceptible to illness and disease. A life full of negativity can predispose us to illness. The negative thoughts, the emotional stress, the sadness – it all makes us acidic, toxic and fat. High stress can lead to high blood pressure, heart disease, and stroke. So what are you waiting for? Are you going to let stress and anxiety take over your life and your body?

Resting easy is not easy for most

Sleep is a critical physiological function and lack of respect for sleep is likely to keep you from living to your full mental potential in addition to predisposing you to disease. Getting rest is important down to the cellular level. Most of us wake up to an alarm clock, rush to work, stress, worry, and work all day, rush to get home, eat a meal, and sit in front of the television to watch all the shows we have recorded. Then we go to bed, and repeat the same process, day in and day out.

Why is it important to get good rest? Surveys conducted by the National Sleep Foundation show that at least 40 million Americans suffer from over 70 different sleep disorders and 60% of adults report having sleep problems a few nights a week or more. Good sleep strengthens your immune system and makes you less prone to various illnesses. It reduces stress, tension and anxiety. Proper rest allows your body to relax and without proper rest your body does not rejuvenate, because your cells are not given the opportunity to recharge. In addition, tired cells cannot eliminate toxins efficiently and we know the importance of detoxification. Simply put, there are three elements of proper rest:

- The time in which you rest
- The amount of hours you rest
- The rest and sleep should be deep

The timeframe from 10pm to 6am allows the body to rest the deepest, rejuvenate the most, and give the person the most energy throughout the day. The hormones that heal the body are released only between 10pm and 2am, and they are only released when the body is in a deep sleep. Try to get to bed by 10pm at least 3 to 4 times per week; we know you will feel the difference. Is the evening news really that important? You can always record it or look up the weather and the sports scores on the internet the next day.

The importance of movement

One of our patients made it very clear that she wanted nothing to do with colonics to clear out her majorly congested colon. We told her if she was not going to consider colonics to clear out her toxins she should at least consider sitting in an infrared sauna to sweat them out. She even resisted this because she did not like breaking a sweat; that was too disgusting for her. Then she found out that sitting in an infrared sauna and sweating for 30-40 minutes was the equivalent of running 8-9 miles. We cannot get her out of the sauna. She is now doing this treatment at least 2 times a week, loving it and finally starting to rid herself of constipation and those last few pounds she had been trying to lose.

In our program we don't emphasis exercise as much as we do movement. Moving the body can mean many things such as breathing deeply, stretching, walking (even in place) and breaking a sweat by sitting in an infrared sauna.

- Movement, no matter how simple, increases oxygen to your cells
- Movement stimulates cells and cell development
- Movement opens energy channels
- Movement helps to release tension and stress
- Movement to the point of breaking a sweat helps to enhance the pumping of your lymphatic system, which in turn removes toxins and acids from tissue and fluid and releases them through your skin

We know the benefit of movement and exercise so why is it so hard to do these things regularly? Movement and exercise like everything else takes time and it takes energy. These are two things most of us do not have a lot of these days. We are so busy with everything else we do not make it a priority and because of our diets we find ourselves with little energy to do anything more than just get through the day.

The groups of people who actually do exercise on and off get their gym memberships and show up to run on the treadmill, use the elliptical, lift weights, etc. They get bored easily with the same routine and when they do not see the results they quit for a while before starting back up again. We are a society of instant gratification and if we do not see results within a few weeks we get discouraged and quit. How many times have you paid for a gym membership only to drive by the gym for months without attending?

Then there are those people who have not moved their body or exercised in years, sometimes decades. It has been such a long time for these individuals that they do not even know where to start. Really what it comes down to is they do not know what options are available to them to start slowly and methodically. No matter what group you fit into there are ideas for helping you put together a movement plan that will stick.

So now that you have learned what is causing your issues, especially your digestive health issues, let's figure out how to solve them.

The #1 solution to digestive issues

The quickest and easiest way to solve a majority of digestive issues comes in the form of digestive enzymes. Digestive enzymes are a collection of important molecules without which we would have a difficult time absorbing our food. Enzymes start in the mouth and follow through the whole digestive process. There is not just one enzyme that breaks down all the food we eat; there are several enzymes that have very specific functions. Without the proper enzymes to fully digest their food you will end up with undigested food in your system wreaking all sorts of havoc and causing symptoms such as gas, bloating, acid reflux, constipation, and diarrhea.

Ironically enough, enzyme development is hindered by lack of proper nutrition and age as our enzyme production decreases over time. This means if you are not eating a nutritious diet to begin with you are limiting your production of enzymes and as you get older the situation worsens. This is usually why we can eat whatever we want as a child but as soon as we get into our 20's or 30's we start having issues. A very simple solution that has solved digestive issues for hundreds of our patients that continue to come back for more is supplementing throughout the day with a digestive enzyme pill with meals.

As opposed to being on medication, many patients decide to try digestive enzymes and realize it is so much better for them then taking a prescription or non-prescription drug. With digestive enzymes there are no side effects or issues with long term use. A digestive enzyme is literally just replacing what the body should be creating on its own.

A plan for life-long digestive health

Digestive enzymes are only the first step toward life-long digestive health. Although they are the very simple answer to many digestive issues there are so many other things to teach you about that can affect your body's digestive process. One thing that shocked me the most as we have been teaching people about digestive wellness is that although all of our bodies technically work the same, no two people react exactly the same to our teachings.

We may have two people present with the exact same symptoms that they have had for the same exact amount of time. We introduce our concepts to them and one thing works for one of them while something totally different works for the other. You never know which bit of knowledge we teach is going to change your life so it is important to learn and try everything to see what is going to work for you.

It is also important to know that the things we teach are not something to incorporate in your life for a short period of time and then stop them once you get the results you are looking for. This is not a get healthy quick scheme. We are teaching you concepts for life – things to live by, for as long as you are living on this earth. Many of you know it is not easy to change habits, especially bad ones, especially ones that surround what we eat and drink and how we live on a daily basis. These are habits that have been ingrained in us since we were children.

We are not only going to have to give you the knowledge you need to help make healthier decisions for your life but we are also going to have to provide life-long support and guidance to help you stick with it. As two people who want to live a healthy life, we know how hard it is to do so day in and day out. Even we falter, especially when we encounter times of stress. The support and guidance is almost if not more important than the knowledge itself. With that being said, let us go into some detail on both, starting with the knowledge you will need.

The knowledge

Tina and I have spent the last few years focused mostly on the knowledge, imparting on others what it took us years to learn and incorporate into our own life. Let me be very clear that what we teach are very simple steps that can be learned on your own; however, wouldn't it be nice to save three years of your life and countless hours of trial and error and just cut to the chase?

After much thought and effort we decided to put our knowledge into an online home study program that we call the "DNA for Digestive Health." We call it the DNA because the DNA of the body represents the core structure of the body and we believe our teachings are the core structure for having true digestive health. The DNA also describes our teaching topics extremely well:

D = Detoxification and Digestive Restoration
N = Nourishment and Necessary Hydration
A = Activating Mind, Body, Soul & Action Plan

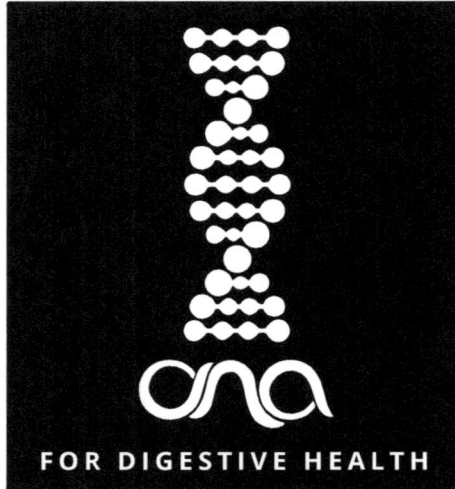

Let me expand on each of these topics a bit to give you some ideas of what you can learn through this online home-study program.

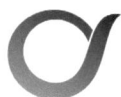

Detoxification is the first topic we teach about because you cannot have healthy digestion with a toxic body. You have to clean out the house first before you start bringing in new furniture. We discuss what detoxification is, why it is so important and the seven best ways to detoxify the body. We also provide several key resources and products so you can work through the steps to detoxify yourself.

There are so many stories we could tell about how detoxification alone cured digestive issues but there are two stories that stand out the most. We had a patient with irritable bowel syndrome (IBS), who had tried everything. We ran all the tests but found nothing medically wrong. IBS can be difficult to treat because it is difficult to find the root cause. We encouraged this patient to try a simple ten day detox kit. These kits (if you find the right one), are merely pills and powders that you take while living your normal life. I say "if you find the right one" because believe me there are some detox kits available today that are very hard on the body.

This patient was very hesitant to do the kit because she was already dealing with bouts of constipation and diarrhea and she did not want to worsen the symptoms she already had. We told her to at least try it and after a day or two if it was making things worse to stop all together. Once she did the kit she was amazed at how it regulated her bowel movements and took away the cramping and bloating. She asked how often she could do one of these kits and we told her no more than one every three months. As you can imagine she is in our office every three months buying another kit.

The second story is about a patient who had been feeling pain in her upper abdomen for the past five years. She underwent extensive testing and evaluation without any cause being found. One of the strategies Tina suggested to her included several sessions of colon hydrotherapy. She was too nervous to try it so we did everything else on her – detoxification supplements, change in diet, water intake, movement etc. Although she felt better in other ways the pain in her abdomen was still not going away. We told her to at least try the colon hydrotherapy and if she did not like it the first time she never had to go back again. After she had her first, she signed up for seven more. After her fifth one she called Tina and started crying, saying that she dumped mud out of her colon the whole session and for the first time in five years she had no pain in her abdomen. These are the stories that cause us to want to heal the world of digestive issues.

The second topic under D is focused on Digestive Restoration. Most of what you read in this book is what we teach for this topic. How the digestive system works and what it needs to function properly. What digestive enzymes are and why they are so important. We also teach a lot about probiotics, what they are and why they are so important to include in your digestive health regimen. We have hundreds of patients on digestive enzymes and probiotics on a daily basis and they do not have to come in to see me anymore for their digestive issues. I would rather see my patients on these supplements than on prescription and non-prescription drugs for the rest of their lives.

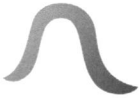

This category of teachings is probably the most important of all. Without nourishment and necessary hydration our bodies cannot function properly. So although the "D" is the first step to digestive health, the "N" is the most important step. There is so much to teach about Nourishment it is difficult to know where to start. We touch on the issues with the food industry which is a lot of what we discussed in this book but then we go into great detail on how to read food labels properly so you can learn how to avoid chemicals, preservatives and sugar as much as possible.

We teach about genetically modified organisms (GMO's) in our food and why they are so important to avoid. We discuss why eating green is so important and how to do it easily at every meal if you wanted to. We have a whole section on why fast food, meat and dairy are wreaking havoc on your digestive system and what the healthier alternatives are to every single thing you consume on a daily basis. We have videos teaching you how to shop for everything from canned goods to vegetables and bread, in addition to videos on how to prepare foods in a healthy way.

We've had so many individuals and families from all walks of life come through our door to learn better ways of eating. When they incorporate our teachings slowly and with baby steps they see amazing results very quickly. More energy, no more digestive issues, and sleeping better are just a few of the many responses we have received from people who have changed their eating habits for good.

The second topic within the "N" category is Necessary Hydration. This should definitely not be overlooked because of the two "N" topics this is the one that makes the most impact on people by far. We teach why water is so important to the body and how much water you should be drinking per day. We also help people understand why not all water is created equal and what type of water you should be drinking. We also discuss and provide products that should be added to your water to truly replenish the body of what it is losing on a daily basis.

Again, patients say that of everything we teach, this topic makes the biggest impact on how they feel. Hundreds of patients have reported no more digestive issues, more energy, less fatigue, more regular bowel movements, no more skin issues, etc. just by drinking the right amount of the right kind of water.

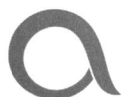

This category of teaching takes digestive health to the next level. By incorporating mind, body and soul into the equation it allows people to take the teachings full circle and incorporate it in every aspect of their life. We discuss some of these topics in this book – stress, rest and movement. From a stress standpoint we discuss how to deal with it properly because let's admit it, in our society it would be hard to teach people to completely eliminate stress. If we have learned anything about people is that everyone is stressed out about something. Even if there is nothing to be stressed about our mind makes stuff up. For some reason our body loves to be in a state of stress all the time. For this reason we teach about how to handle it not necessarily how to eliminate it.

With regard to rest we go into detail on why it is so important to get good rest and what the best ways are to get a good night's sleep. We also go into painstaking detail about the lymphatic system, most people don't know they have a lymphatic system and the ones that do know, do not have any idea what it does. So we teach about why it is important to know about your lymphatic system and how to move your body to keep it clean and doing its job for you. We also teach about deep breathing and the positive affects it has on your digestive health. When was the last time you took a deep breath? Take one now and see how good it feels.

We have had dozens of patients turn their digestive issues around, get off of sleep medications and even lose weight from following the teachings from this topic. Everything we teach is so simple yet it can literally transform your life and your digestive health. The only challenge is finding the one or two things that make the biggest difference for you.

The final step in the *"DNA for Digestive Health"* is the Action Plan. You will learn how to take everything you learned and put it into a three month, six month and nine month plan. This step in the process is very important because without writing in down in the Action Plan Workbook it is very difficult to incorporate your plan into your life. You have to write it down in order for it to happen. Dozens of patients have admitted that without the plan the knowledge is meaningless.

The other thing to know about this step is that it is very important to take baby steps and do things very methodically. We teach you how to do this effectively for lasting change. It is not a race, it took you years to get where you are and it is okay if it takes months or years to get where you want to be. All that matters is you get there, it is never too late to turn the body around.

In addition to walking you through how to create the plan for yourself, we also teach you what to expect once you begin turning the body around, tips for healthy eating while travelling and tips for how to share your knowledge with others. Let's face it, you are going to be looking and feeling better than ever and people are going to start asking you what you are doing different. You are going to have to be prepared to share the knowledge yourself.

The support and guidance

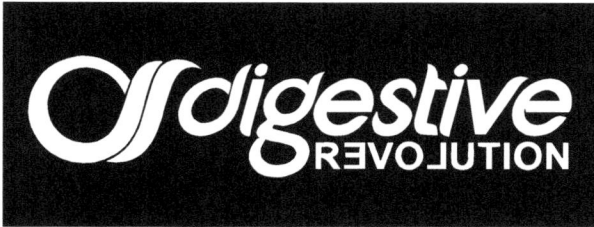

In addition to the ***"DNA for Digestive Health"*** we also created a website called **www.digestiverevolution.com.** This is your resource to help support and guide you through the program and every day thereafter. This is an online community of like-minded people who are all working through the same life transformation and are there to support each other. In addition, this is where Tina and I spend most of our time, helping those that are serious about life-long digestive health.

We realize that without support and guidance it is easy to falter. It is really hard to stick to something new when we have no one to be accountable to and we have no one to share our successes or struggles with. We all need constant reminders for why following the ***"DNA for Digestive Health"*** is so critical to our life-long digestive health.

The website provides the following resources:

- Access to an exclusive Digestive Revolution Facebook page for support and guidance from Dr. Cruz, Tina and fellow members
- An ability to submit and search for recipes, movies, restaurants, and services
- Access to monthly motivational calls where we will highlight one success story each month
- Reminders, general tips, and travel tips
- An advanced frequently asked question section
- Common excuses and how to overcome them
- Special / exclusive product or service offerings not offered to anyone else

It is meant to be a community of love and support to help us all work toward our goals of true digestive health.

Why investing in your health is so important

We tend to invest in everything else except our health. We unfortunately don't think about our health unless we are sick, by then you will pay any amount of money to get well. The reality is you will spend the money one way or another, either on doctor's bills, medicines, surgeries and co-pays or on preventative care, healthy food and water. There are two questions you need to ask yourself:

1. **What's the cost of not feeling well on a regular basis?**

   *   Aside from the money aspect of doctor's bills, deductibles, medicines, etc.; what about losing time with family and friends, or missing work and possibly not getting paid. It is very difficult when your life revolves around doctor's appointments and medicines you need to take.
   *   There is nothing fun about being sick or having aches and pains all the time. Many of my patients cannot even remember what it feels like to be pain free. How sad is that, living a life in pain all the time when there are real solutions that can make you feel better right now.
   *   Aren't you tired of trying every doctor, every drug and things only seem to get worse? At what point are you going to say to yourself this strategy is not working, it is time to try something different?

2. **What would life be like without your digestive issues?**

   *   Close your eyes and imagine your life without your digestive symptoms or issues. How do you feel? What are you able to do that you could not do yesterday? How is your life different? How is your time spent differently?
   *   It truly is time to take matters into your own hands and take back your health.
   *   Knowing how much you have spent on everything else, how could you not make the investment in your future well being?

But Dr. Cruz...what if?

I cannot tell you the excuses we hear from patients who need a major transformation in their digestive health but try to figure out any reason why not to move forward. Below are the top four excuses we hear all the time and how I respond every time.

1. **I do not have time right now to do this.**

   That is why we make it a home study program so you can do it whenever it is convenient for you from the comfort of your own home. Even if you want to start it 2 or 3 months from now you can, all the materials will be there when you are ready.

2. **I do not have the money right now.**

   Think about all the money you have spent and will continue to spend on doctors, deductibles, medicines, etc. If you truly want to get well you cannot afford not to do this. Plus we tend to find the money for things that are a priority for us. For example not having the money to purchase a colonics session but finding a way to buy the new television you have been wanting. If your excuse in the end is that you do not have the money, have you prioritized getting well?

3. **My spouse will not be supportive.**

   Your spouse may be part of the reason you are in this situation to begin with. If you know you need a major transformation and they do not feel the same, please do not let them hold you back. We have plenty of resources and tools to support you along the way without them cheering you on. And let me ask you something, if your car was broken down right now and you had to invest $995 to get it fixed would your spouse support you? Of course they would…yet when it comes to our own body we refuse to invest in its well being… why is that?

4. **I do not trust myself to do the work.**

   If you cannot trust yourself to sit in front of a computer once a week to learn something new or be on a phone call with me once per month and follow my instructions as I show you exactly how to transform your digestive health, it is probably best if you do not do this program. But if you are ready to have a breakthrough in this area and this is calling you, we welcome you.

My recommendation to you

Day in and day out I see patients in consultation for their digestive health issues. Usually it is to set them up for labs, imaging studies or endoscopic procedures. If you are having digestive issues and have never been worked up by a Gastroenterologist I do suggest taking the time to do this, mainly to make sure you do not have something seriously wrong with you.

If all of your tests come back normal and you are dealing with ongoing symptoms that cannot be explained, my recommendation is a lot simpler and will hopefully cost you a lot less time and money and may even save you multiple trips to see your doctor(s). That is right, I am telling you I would rather see you healthy than see you in my office. With that being said everyone should know that the world of medicine is changing. I am here to tell you that getting in to see a doctor is going to get harder not easier. It is going to cost more not less for medical care as we move forward these next several years.

My recommendation is get yourself healthy so you do not have to be a victim of our medical system. Take responsibility for your health and the health of your family because no one is going to care about you more than you. I want to give you every tool you can possibly need to do this without doctors and without drugs. Think of the consequences. I hope this book has provided enough knowledge to make you yearn for more – whether you do it alone or do it with me. If you are ready and you want my helping hand along the way follow these next three simple steps to take your current learning to the next level:

1. Go online to **www.drlizcruz.com** and sign up for our free bi-weekly newsletter – in addition to receiving an email every other week from us giving you great digestive health tips you will also receive our list of the Top 10 Movies That Will Change Your Digestive Health. Start watching some of these movies and hopefully it will start changing the way you see the world.

2. While you are on **www.drlizcruz.com** sign-up to take our Online Digestive Health Assessment. It is a 25 question assessment to see where you are on your path to digestive health and based on your results helps to guide you on the best place to start for making changes for the better.

3. Spend a little more time at **www.drlizcruz.com** reading up on The DNA for Digestive Health packages and the Digestive Revolution online community.

We would love to teach you what we know and have you as part of our Digestive Revolution family. Because I want to help you get healthy as fast as possible, below are my high level recommendations for each step in the DNA. There is so much to teach you behind each one of these recommendations but at least it will allow you to get started.

- **Detoxification** – consider our Delicate Detox™ supplement to help rid your body of toxins.

- **Digestive Restoration** – consider our Everyday Enzymes™ and Pleasant Probiotics™ to restore the body's digestive processes to normal working condition.

- **Nutrition** – consider eating more greens on a daily basis, red or green leaf lettuce in salads, steaming bok choy or green swiss chard a couple times per week, or using avocados on toast in the morning instead of butter. Or if you cannot stand eating greens consider taking our Gastro Greens™ supplement to get your dose of greens every day.

- **Necessary Hydration** – consider drinking more water and less of everything else, ideally you want to work up to drinking half of your body weight in ounces per day.

- **Activating the Mind, Body and Soul** – consider walking in place a few minutes each day and going to bed by 10pm at least three times per week.

- **Action Plan** – take the time to write down your goals and plans, it will help you stick with them as much as possible. And when you falter (and you will falter) do not feel bad, just turn it around and get back on track again.

In case you were wondering, Tina and I do speak regularly so if you have an event or a group of people that you think could benefit from this message please let us know by going to **www.drlizcruz.com/learning/speaking**.

In addition, if you or any group you belong to would like to have a "Day with Dr. Cruz" I am available for private sessions. For more information go to **www. drlizcruz.com/learning/daywithdrcruz.**

Here is to a future of life-long digestive health for all!

Liz Cruz M.D.

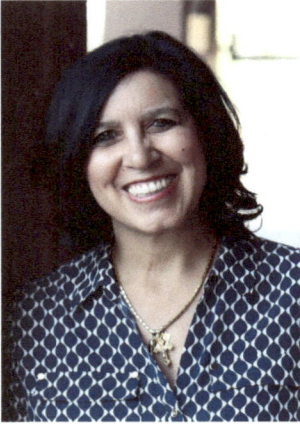

Dr. Cruz graduated from college in 1988 with a B.S. in Medical Technology. Prior to Medical School, she taught English for one year in Bangkok Thailand. In 1989, Dr. Cruz began her formal career in medicine by attending Loma Linda University School of Medicine in California. During medical school, Dr. Cruz was part of a student / staff physician team, which provided relief work to the natives along the Amazon River. She graduated from medical school in 1993 and then went on to do her Internal Medicine Internship under the auspices of the U.S. Navy at the Naval Hospital, Oakland, California.

Upon the closure of the Naval Hospital in Oakland, Dr. Cruz transferred and completed her internal medicine residency at the University of California, San Francisco. In 1996, she was deployed to Guam to fulfill her commitment to the U.S. Navy. While in Guam, she served as a Staff Internist at the U.S. Naval Hospital. During her active duty years in the Navy, she received the Meritorious Unit Commendation Medal as well as the Humanitarian Service Medal and the National Defense Medal for service during Operation Desert Storm. During her last two years in Guam, she was the Head of the Internal Medicine Division at the U.S. Naval Hospital.

In 2000, she went back to the University of California, San Francisco where she completed her training in Gastroenterology (GI). In 2004, Dr. Cruz moved to Arizona to join the Arizona Medical Clinic in Peoria. She served as a full-time gastroenterologist in both the outpatient and inpatient settings doing the full range of general gastroenterology including endoscopic procedures as well as hepatology. In January 2007, she opened the doors to her own practice, Digestive Healthcare Associates, LLC in Phoenix, Arizona.

In 2010, Dr. Cruz along with her life partner, Tina Nunziato began offering the Dr. Liz Cruz Wellness Program to educate patients on the very things that were causing their digestive issues. After helping hundreds of patients improve and in some cases eliminate their digestive issues through detoxification, digestive restoration, nutrition, and proper hydration, Dr. Cruz decided to launch her products and services online. Her *"DNA for Digestive Health"* 3 step program and the www.DigestiveRevolution.com online community she created are changing people's digestive health for good. More information about her products and services can be found at **www.drlizcruz.com** and through her "Digest This™" podcast at **www.digestthispodcast.com**.

Dr. Cruz was born in Los Angeles, California and was raised in Orlando, Florida. She speaks fluent Spanish and enjoys her family, traveling, jazz music, and photography.

Dr. Cruz is a Diplomate of the American Board of Internal Medicine and the American Board of Gastroenterology. She is a member of the American College of Gastroenterology and the American Society for Gastrointestinal Endoscopy.

Tina Nunziato, C.H.N.C.

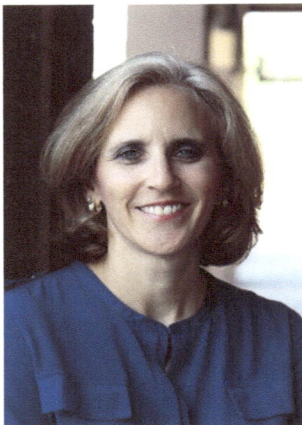

Tina Nunziato graduated from the Arizona State University College of Business Honors Program in 1996 with a Bachelor of Science in Marketing. While attending ASU she was very active in the College of Business and the Residence Hall Association. As the College of Business Honors Program Marketing Coordinator, Ms. Nunziato worked for four years creating programs for Honors students that still exist today. As the President for the Residence Hall Association, Ms. Nunziato worked with other student organizations to better the life of all campus residents.

After graduation Ms. Nunziato took her first job out of college as a Marketing Analyst for a local telecommunications vendor, now Lucent Technologies. She quickly moved out of market research and into business development as a Marketing Specialist where she worked on various new product and joint venture initiatives. In addition, Ms. Nunziato was also responsible for managing projects produced by the students at Thunderbird Graduate School of Management.

In late 1999, during the dot-com boom, Ms. Nunziato moved to San Francisco to start a web-based software company with a fellow ASU College of Business graduate. Focused on the park and recreation market, the company went through many strategy iterations before it found its niche. In her role as COO and eventually CEO, Ms. Nunziato experienced all facets of business from raising capital and product design to selling, training and supporting customers. In May of 2003, subsequent to selling her company to one of the industry competitors, Ms. Nunziato came back to her roots here in Arizona. After rebuilding her network and consulting for various companies to determine her next step, she accepted a position with Carefx Corporation, a healthcare software company in Scottsdale. As the Director of Marketing, Ms. Nunziato was responsible for all marketing initiatives including corporate and product messaging, sales tool development, managing strategic planning, and all print, web and tradeshow initiatives. Ms. Nunziato resigned from Carefx in 2006 to pursue Consult TNT with her father.

In 2007 Ms. Nunziato decided to try her hand in medicine when she started Digestive Healthcare Associates, LLC with her life and business partner Dr. Elizabeth Cruz. In addition to having a successful Gastroenterology practice Ms. Nunziato and Dr. Cruz took medicine one step further by offering a wellness program through their office. In conjunction with and to support this business Ms. Nunziato went back to school to receive her Certificate in Holistic Nutrition in 2010. Since then both businesses have been growing as they continue to heal patients year after year from digestive disease, sluggishness and weight gain.

It is the passion of both Ms. Nunziato and Dr. Cruz to get the digestive wellness message to as many people as possible as fast as possible so to help heal a nation.

Resources

Hundreds of books were read between myself and Tina throughout our educational process. Some of the teachings in this book came from the following resources:

- 7-Day Detox Miracle – by Peter Bennett, N.D. and Stephen Barrie, N.D.
- Cellular Cleansing Made Easy – by Scott Ohlgren
- Colon Health – by Dr. Norman Walker
- Sugar Blues – by William Dufty
- The Acid Alkaline Balance Diet – by Felicia Drury Kliment
- The Acid – Alkaline Diet for Optimum Health – by Christopher Vasey, N.D.
- The Acid Alkaline Food Guide – by Dr. Susan Brown and Larry Trivieri, Jr.
- The pH Miracle Balance Your Diet, Reclaim Your Health – by Robert O. Young, PhD and Shelley Redford Young
- The pH Miracle for Weight Loss – by Robert O. Young, PhD and Shelley Redford Young
- Tissue Cleansing Through Bowel Management – by Bernard Jensen, D.C., PhD, Nutritionist
- Toxic Relief – by Don Colbert, M.D.
- Why Our Health Matters – by Andrew Weil, M.D.